PREFACE

I0484934

My name is Valencia Annik Payne, BSN, RN, BS, Biology. I received my BS in Nursing from Delta State University and my BS in Biology from Jackson State University. I am a former Navy PACU RN that has instructed and tutored many nursing students, as well as, many Registered Nurses. As the Author of Fluid and Electrolytes for Nursing Students and Dimensional Analysis for Nursing Students now comes GI for Nursing Students. In the nursing profession, it not about learning one concept but all concepts as this will provide positive patient outcomes. Please enjoy this colorful and exemplary learning tool.

CONTENTS

CIRRHOSIS

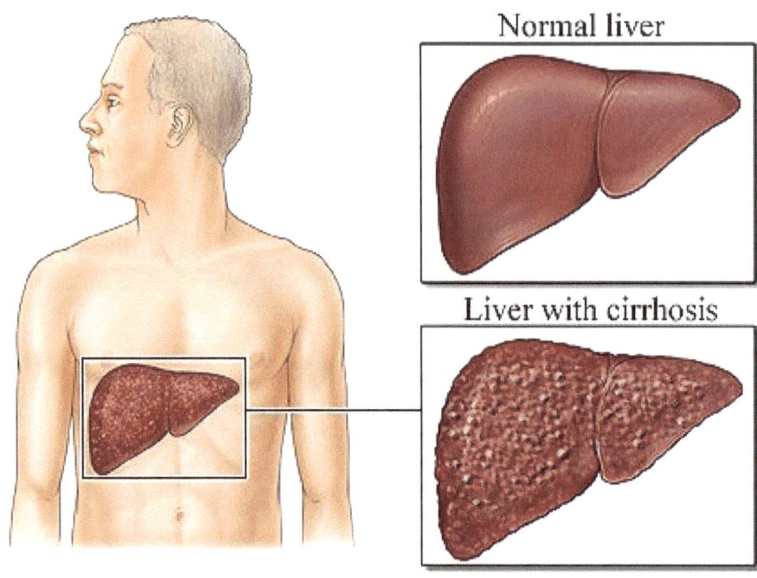

Normal liver

Liver with cirrhosis

A. Scarring of the liver and poor liver function. It is the final phase of chronic liver disease

B. Portal Hypertension: Liver cells are destroyed and are replaced with scar connective tissue which alters the circulation within the liver. This causes the blood pressure in the liver to elevate

SIGNS AND SYMPTOMS

A. Firm liver

B. Abdominal pain

C. Change in bowel habits

D. Ascites

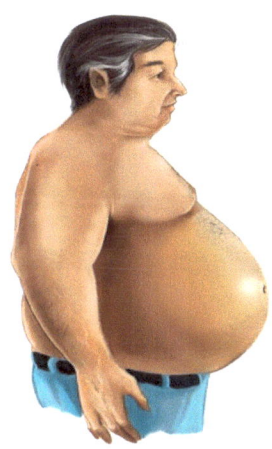

E. Chronic dyspepsia

F. Splenomegaly: Immune system is in overdrive

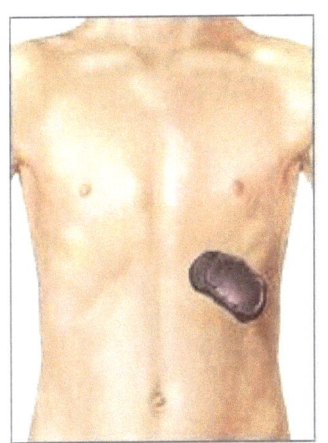
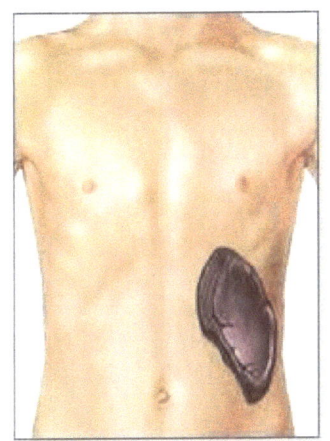

Normal spleen   Splenomegaly

G. Decrease serum albumin.

H. Increased SGOT & SGPT

I. Anemia

It will progress to hepatic encephalopathy/coma. Why: Ammonia has a sedative effect

TREATMENT

A. No Alcohol!!

B. I & O and daily weights (When you have ascites then there is a fluid volume issue)

C. Antacids, diuretics, and vitamins

D. Rest

E. Bleeding Precautions

F. Measure abdominal girth

G. Monitor jaundice (Check Sclera)

H. Avoid Narcotics Why: Liver cannot metabolize the drugs

DIET

A. Low sodium diet

B. Decrease protein

HEPATIC COMA

A. When the liver becomes impaired, it cannot make this conversion. Therefore, ammonia builds up in the bloodstream.

SIGNS AND SYMPTOMS

A. Asterixis: Hand tremor or "liver flap"

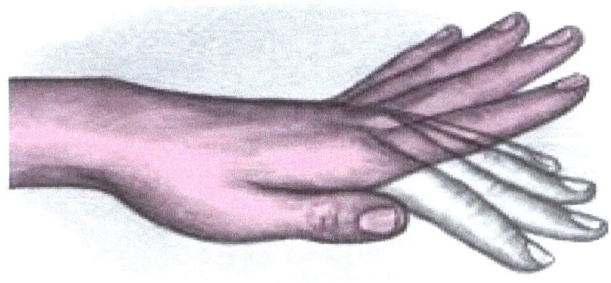

Recognizing asterixis

In asterixis, the patient's wrists and fingers are observed to "flap" because of a brief, rapid relaxation of wrist dorsiflexion.

B. Handwriting changes: 1st sign of liver problem

C. Reflexes are decreased

D. Difficulty awakening

E. Minor mental changes/motor problems

F. Fetor: Also known as Breath of the Dead or Ammonia Breath (It is a sweet fecal smell and it is a late sign in liver failure

G. EEG: Slow

TREATMENT

A. Neomycin Sulfate (decrease ammonia-producing bacteria in the gut)

B. Cleansing enemas: Decreases NH_3^+

C. Lactulose (decrease serum ammonia)

D. Decrease protein in the diet

E. Monitor serum ammonia

BLEEDING ESOPHAGEAL VARICES

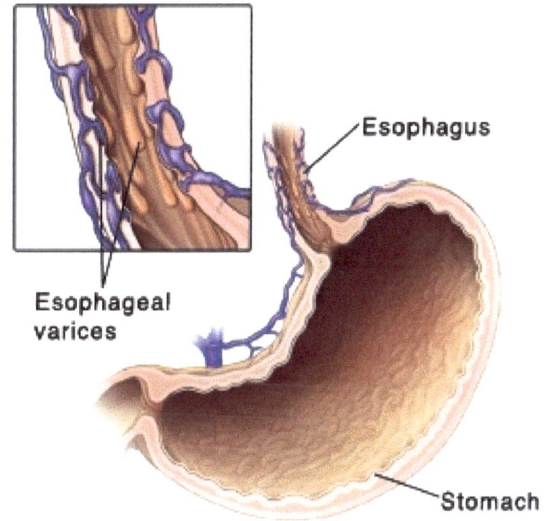

A. Due to Portal Hypertension (High blood pressure in the liver), forces the formation of collateral circulation (New circulation)

This collateral circulation forms in 3 places (Esophagus, Stomach, & Rectum)

1. When you see an alcoholic client that has gastrointestinal bleeding and is usually due to collateral circulation. Normally it is not a problem until rupture.

TREATMENT

A. Replace blood loss

B. Vital signs (Maintain)

C. O2 (Due to being anemic)

D. MgSO42- (Magnesium sulfate) enema flushes any blood out

E. Neomycin: Decreases ammonia producing bacteria

F. Sandostatin: Lowers BP in the liver

G. Sengstaken Blakemore Tube: Hold pressure on bleeding varices

To reestablish airway: CUT THE TUBE

H. Saline lavage: Get blood out of the stomach

PANCREATITIS

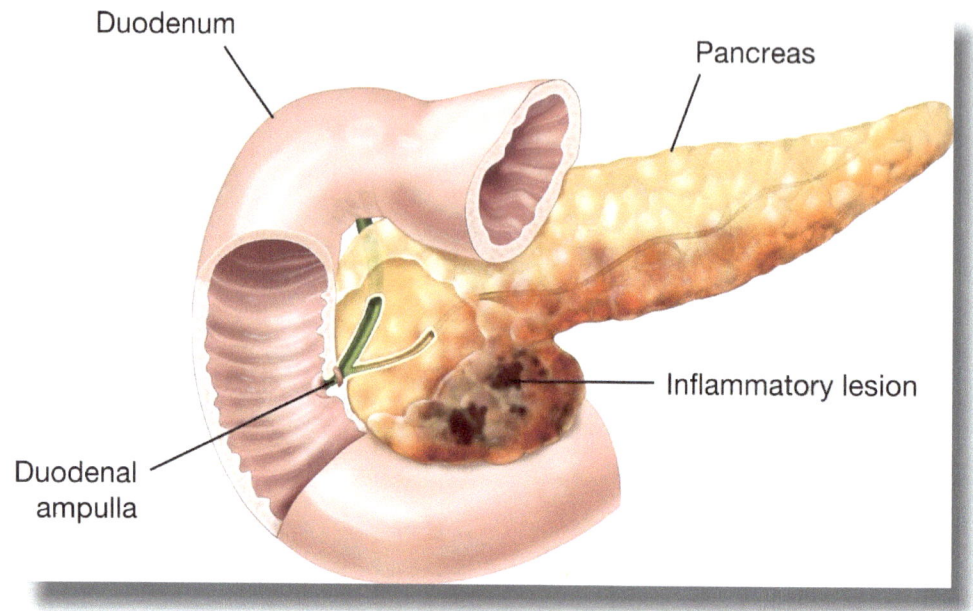

A. In pancreatitis, pancreatic enzymes become activated and begin to auto-digest the pancreas

B. Autodigestion of the pancreas

C. Enzymes activate in the small intestines

FUNCTIONS OF THE PANCREAS

A. Endocrine: Insulin

B. Exocrine: Digestive enzymes

TYPES OF PANCREATITIS

A. Acute (Caused by alcohol & gallbladder disease)

B. Chronic (Caused by alcohol)

DIAGNOSTIC TEST

A. ERCP (Endoscopic retrograde cholangiopancreatogram): Allows the doctor to see the structure of the common bile duct, other bile ducts, &the pancreatic duct. The only diagnostic test used to treat narrow areas (strictures) of the bile ducts & remove gallstones from the common bile duct

SIGNS AND SYMPTOMS

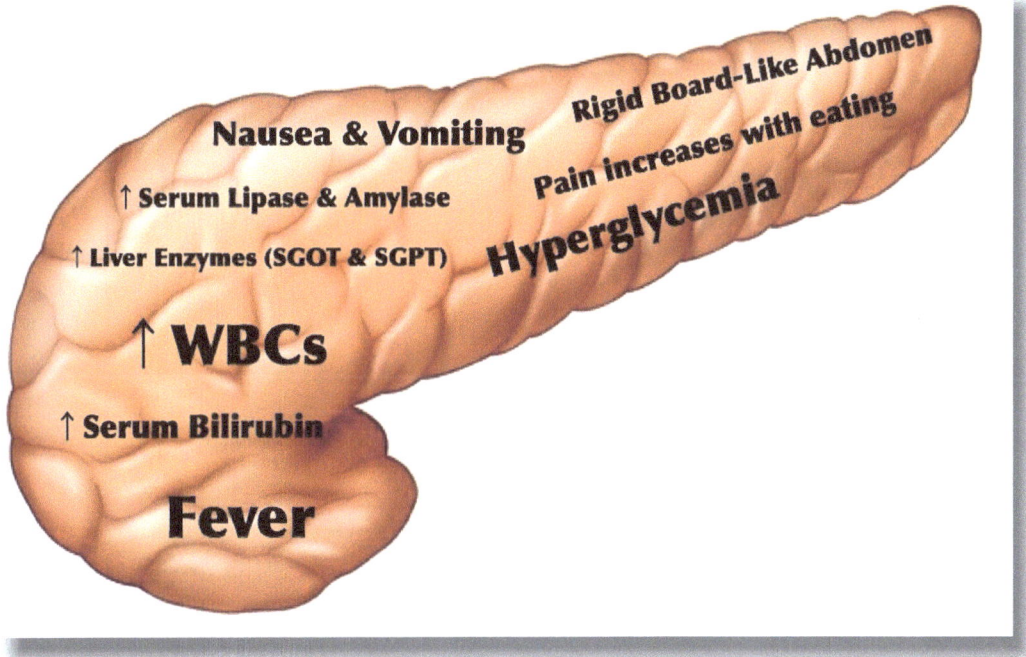

A. Abdominal distention (Ascites)

Why: Because circulating pancreatic enzymes damages capillaries causing ASCITES

B. Bruising

1. Cullen's sign: Ring around the umbilical area

2. Gray Turner's: Ring around the flank area

C. Jaundice: Due to the enzymes eating up the liver

D. Hypotension: Due to bleeding and ascites

E. Elevated hemoglobin and hematocrit: Due to dehydration

TREATMENT

A. Decrease gastric secretions (Bed rest, NPO, NGT to suction)

a. Why: Because you want the stomach empty and dry

B. Demerol is the DRUG OF CHOICE

C. Fentanyl patches, Dilaudid, PCA Narcotics, & Toradol

DO NOT USE MORPHINE Why: It causes spasm of the sphincter of oddi (Muscle that surrounds the exit of the bile duct and pancreatic duct into the duodenum)

D. Steroids: Keeps down inflammation but the glucose level increases. Give insulin to decrease the glucose levels caused by steroids

E. Maintain fluid and electrolyte balance

ULCERATIVE COLITIS AND CROHN'S DISEASE

A. Ulcerative colitis: Ulcerative inflammatory bowel disease

ONLY IN THE LARGE INTESTINE

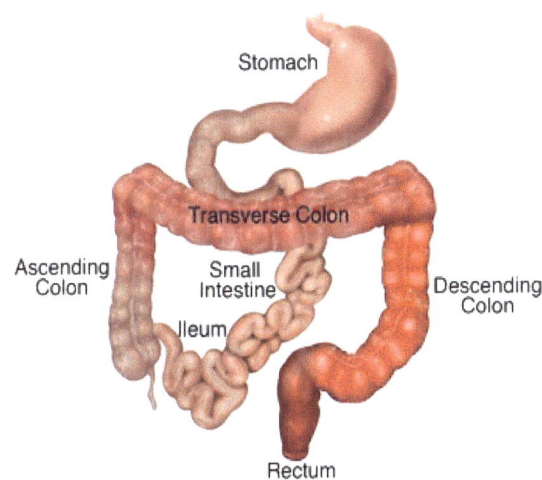

B. Crohn's Disease: Inflammation & erosion of the ileum

CAN BE FOUND ANYWHERE

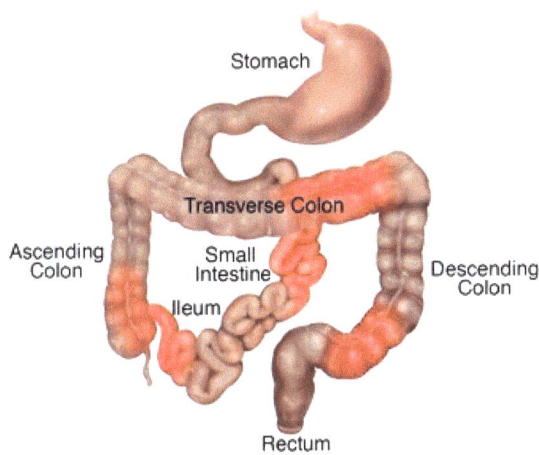

SIGNS AND SYMPTOMS

A. Diarrhea

B. Rectal bleeding

C. Weight loss

D. Vomiting

E. Cramping

F. Dehydration

G. Blood in stools

H. Anemic

I. Rebound tenderness (Peritoneal inflammation)

J. Fever

TREATMENT

A. Low fiber: Trying to limit motility to help save fluid

B. Avoid cold & hot foods & smoking: These increase motility

C. Antibiotics: Sulfonamides

D. Steroids

E. Anti-diarrheals: Give them for symptomatically mild ulcerative colitis ONLY

SURGERY

A. Ulcerative colitis

1. Kock's Pouch or J Pouch (No bag just a valve)

2. Total colectomy (Have an ileostomy)

3. Temporary colostomy: This is the removal of the colon/rectum and the ileum is attached to the anal area

The purpose of a temporary colostomy is to allow the intestines the allotted time needed to rest and heal

B. Crohn's

1. Remove only the affected area

Patient will end up with an ileostomy or a colostomy

OSTOMY CARE

A. Ileostomy care: DO NOT IRRIGATE

1. Continuous fluid drainage

2. Avoid rough foods (Hard to digest)

3. Always a little dehydrated

a. At risk for kidney stones

b. Gatorade in the summer

B. Colostomy Care

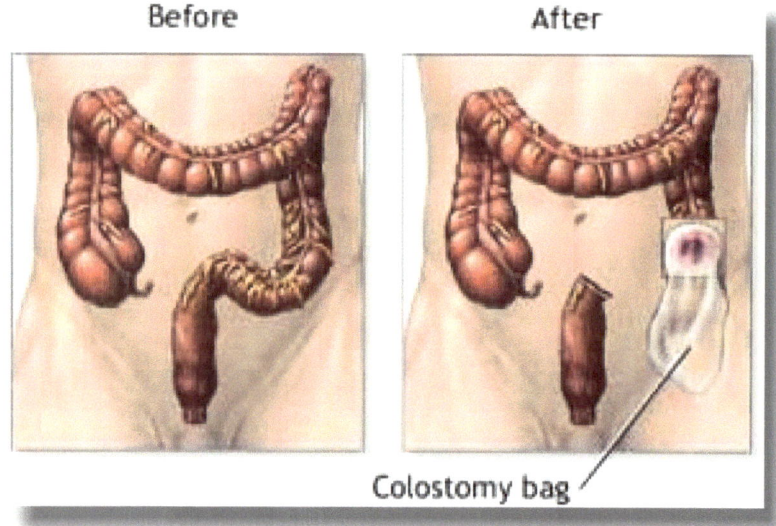

Before   After

Colostomy bag

1. Regulation is through IRRIGATION & BOWEL TRAINING

2. Why or where might we irrigate a colostomy? To establish regularity and evacuation of hard stool

3. When is the best time to irrigate? It is done at the same time everyday and after a meal because you have more peristalsis

AS YOU GO DOWN THE COLON, THE MORE FORMED THE STOOL WILL BECOME BECAUSE WATER IS BEING DRAWN OUT

APPENDICITIS: SCARED OF RUPTURE (Leakage of bowel contents in abdomen)

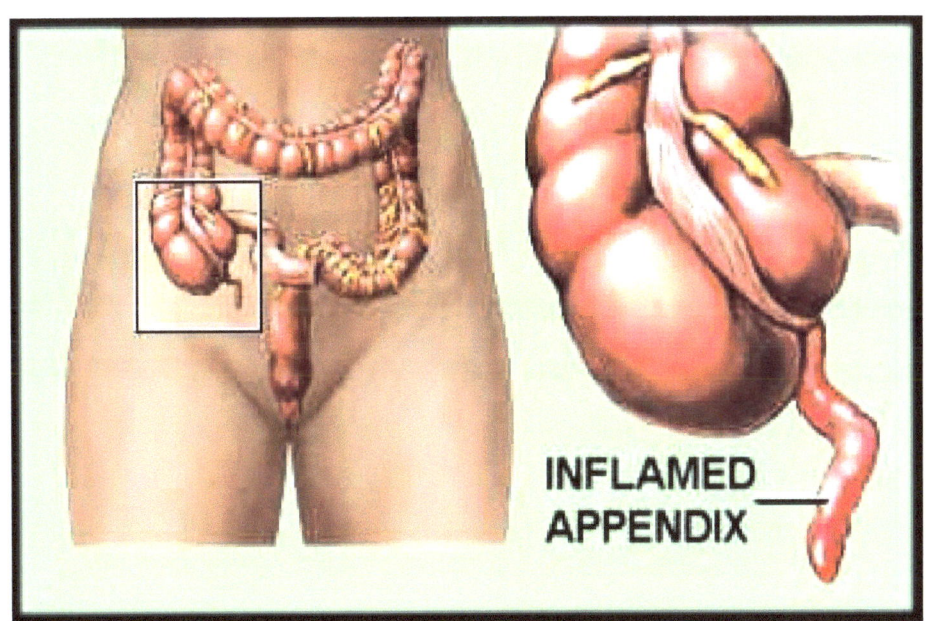

INFLAMED
APPENDIX

A. This is related to low fiber diet

SIGNS AND SYMPTOMS

A. Initially you have generalized pain that will become localized at the McBurney's Point (Right Lower Quadrant)

B. Increase in WBCs

C. Nausea and vomiting

D. Rebound tenderness

E. No enema

F. Laparoscopic surgery is done unless perforation has occurred

Any abdominal surgery SEMI-FOWLER is the position of choice

PEPTIC ULCERS

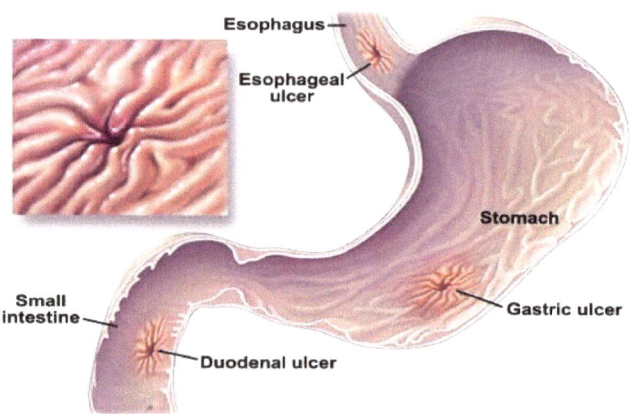

A. Common cause of GI bleeding

B. <u>S</u>am <u>D</u>oes <u>E</u>at (can be in the <u>S</u>tomach, <u>D</u>uodenum, & <u>E</u>sophagus)

C. Occurs mainly in males

D. Erosion is present

SIGNS AND SYMPTOMS

A. Burning pain in the mid-epigastric area

TREATMENT

A. Prilosec, Protonix, Prevacid, & Nexium (Proton pump inhibitors that decrease acid secretions)

B. Zantac and Pepcid

C. Liquid antacids to coat the stomach

TAKE ON EMPTY STOMACH & at bedtime because the stomach is empty and the stomach acid will get on the ulcer. The antacid protects the ulcer

D. Decreases stress

E. Stop smoking

F. Avoid extra spicy foods and caffeine

PEOPLE THAT ARE WORKER BEES GET GASTRIC ULCERS

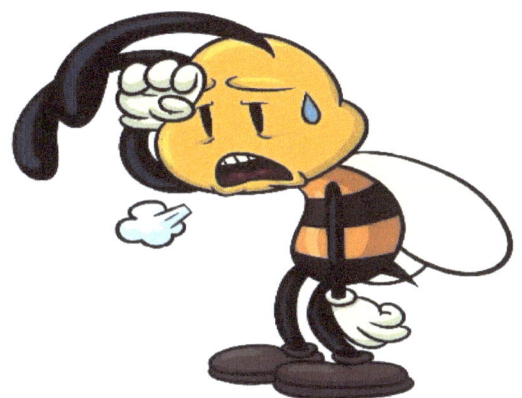

A. Malnourished

B. Pain is usually half hour to one hour after meals

C. Food does not help but vomiting does (Vomit Blood)

PEOPLE THAT ARE PEDIGREES GET DUODENAL ULCERS

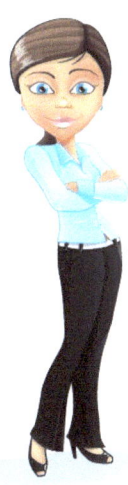

A. Well nourished

B. Common to have night time pain and 2-3 hours after meals

C. Food HELPS

D. Blood in stools

DUMPING SYNDROME

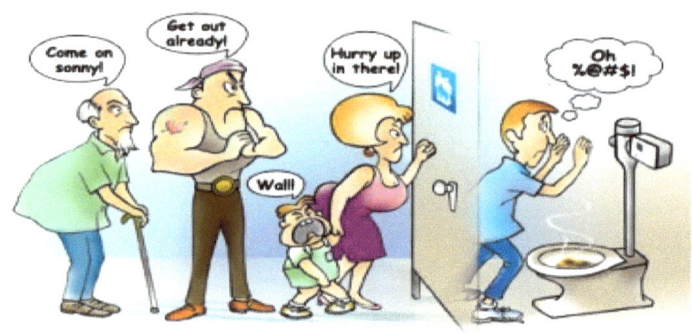

A. The stomach empties too quickly and the patient experiences uncomfortable and severe side effects

SIGNS AND SYMPTOMS

A. Fullness

B. Weakness

C. Palpitations

D. Faintness

E. Cramping

F. Diarrhea

TREATMENT

A. Semi-recumbent with meals

B. No fluids with meals (Drink in-between meals)

C. Lie down after meals on your left side

D. Decrease carb intake because carbs empty fast

HIATAL HERNIA

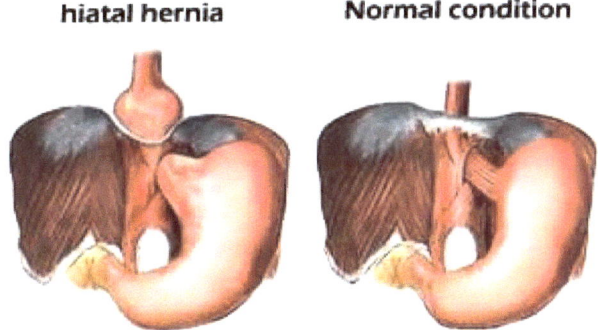

hiatal hernia   Normal condition

A. When the hole in the diaphragm is too large and the stomach moves up into the thoracic cavity

Congenital abnormalities, trauma, and surgery are other causes of hiatal hernia

SIGNS AND SYMPTOMS

A. Heart burn

B. Regurgitation

C. Fullness after eating

D. Dysphagia

TREATMENT

A. Small frequent meals

B. Sit up 1 hour after eating

C. Elevate HOB

D. Surgery

HYPERALIMENTATION

TPN (Total Parenteral Nutrition) 20-50% Glucose

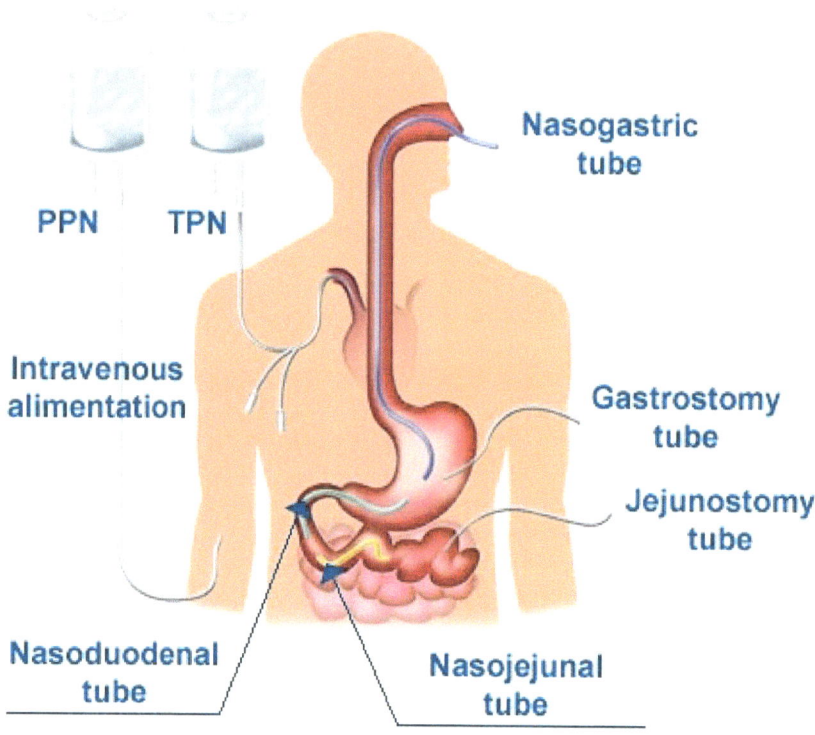

1. Need a filter and a central line because TPN is packed with particles that eat up peripheral veins

2. Keep refrigerated and let it sit out for a few minutes prior to administration

3. Once a port has been selected to infuse the TPN, it should not be changed from that port due to increased risk of infection

4. Discontinue gradually to avoid hypoglycemia

5. Daily weights

6. May have to start taking insulin

7. Check urine for glucose and ketones

8. Can only be hung for 24 hrs.

9. Change tubing with each new bag

10. TPN may be covered with dark bag to prevent chemical breakdown

11. Needs to be on a pump

12. Most frequent complication: INFECTION

13. Accu-checks every 6 hrs

PPN (Peripheral parenteral nutrition) 20% Glucose

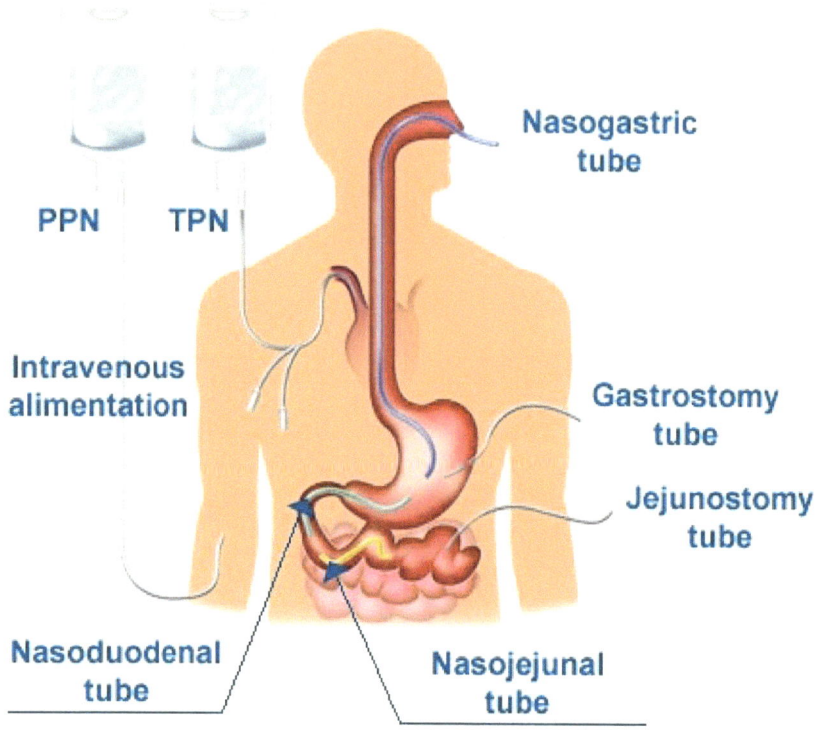

1. Used when additional nutritional support is needed for a short time, the caloric and protein intake is not adequate, or the risk is high to put in a central line

2. Administered through a peripheral IV

3. Phlebitis & volume overload are common complications

A. Upper GI

1. Looks at the esophagus and stomach with dye

2. NPO past midnight

3. No smoking

Smoking increases stomach acid and motility that will affect the test

B. Barium Enema

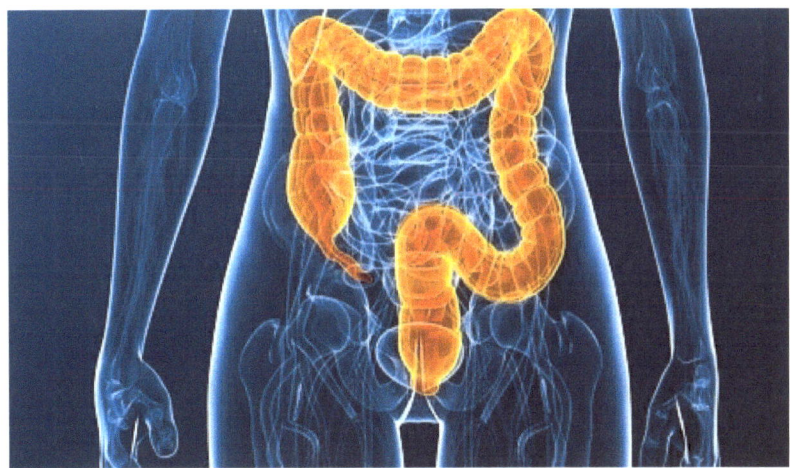

1. Clear liquids

2. Laxative or enemas until clear

3. The client needs a BOWEL MOVEMENT POST-PROCEDURE

C. Gastroscopy (Endoscopy)

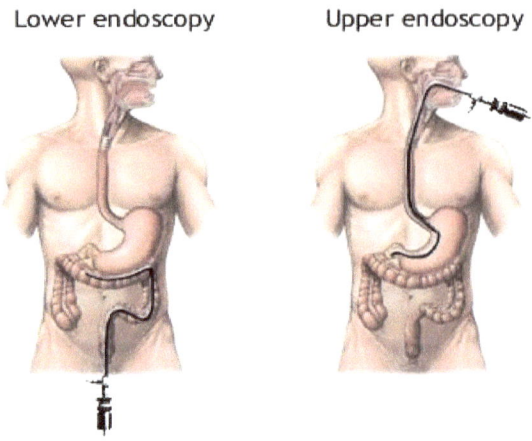

1. NPO pre procedure and post procedure until GAG REFLEX returns

2. Sedated

3. Need to watch for perforation (Unusual discomfort and pain)

D. Liver Biopsy *Liver problems=Bleeding*

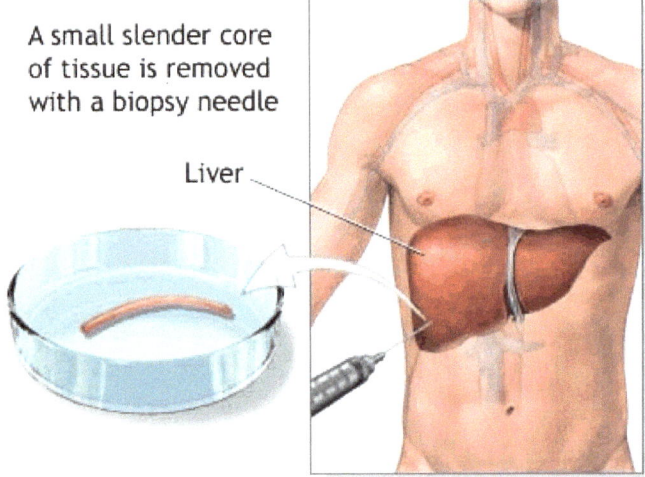

1. Pre-procedure clotting studies

2. Position client during procedure supine with right arm behind head

3. Exhale & hold (This gets the diaphragm out of the way)

4. Post procedure: Lie on right side

5. Main function of the liver: Detoxifies the body, helps to clot blood, metabolizes drugs, and synthesizes albumin

E. Paracentesis

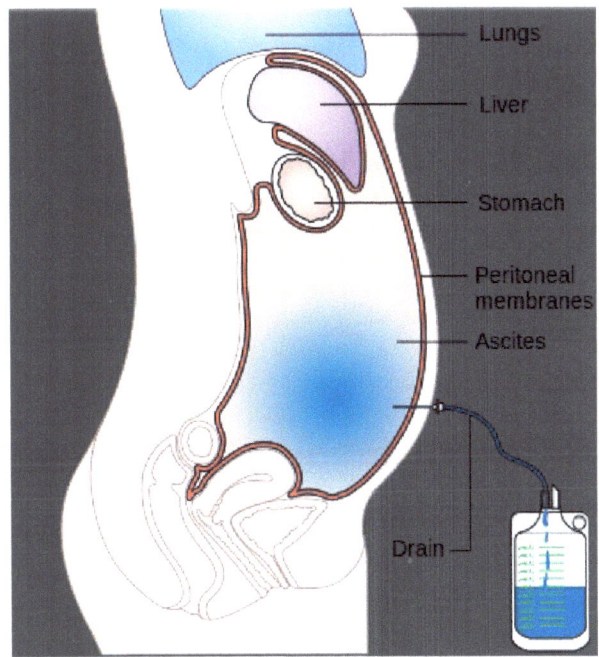

Labels in figure: Lungs, Liver, Stomach, Peritoneal membranes, Ascites, Drain

1. Removal of fluid from the peritoneal cavity (ascites)

2. Have patient to void

3. Position upright

NCLEX PRACTICE QUESTIONS

1. During a hospital admission assessment, a nurse suspects GERD (gastrointestinal reflux disease) when the client says:

A. I have been having night sweats

B. I feel sleepy after meals

C. At night, I wake up with a burning feeling in my chest

D. I get headaches after meals

2. A client has Zenker's diverticulum. What is the priority nursing diagnosis?

A. Altered nutrition related to dysphagia

B. Risk for aspiration related to regurgitation of accumulated food in the diverticula

C. Pain related to GERD

D. Constipation related to sigmoid colon changes

3. A client with esophageal cancer underwent an esophagectomy. The client is beginning to eat solid foods. The nurse is concerned that the client may aspirate because the client no longer has:

A. Pharynx

B. Pyloric sphincter

C. Stomach

D. Lower esophageal sphincter

NCLEX ANSWERS

1. **C is correct**

Rationale: The most common symptom of GERD is heartburn.

2. **B is correct**

Rationale: The outpouching of the esophagus near the hypopharyngeal sphincter is the Zenker's diverticulum. This is where food becomes trapped and causes aspiration.

3. **D is correct**

Rationale: An esophagectomy is the removal of the lower esophageal sphincter. In normal cases, the esophageal sphincter keeps the food from refluxing back into the esophagus.

DOWNLOAD THE APP

REFERENCES

Berkowitz, A. (2007). *Clinical pathophysiology made ridiculously simple*. Miami, FL: MedMaster Inc.

Ignatavicius, D., & Workman, M. (2006). *Medical-Surgical Nursing critical thinking for collaborative care*. Saint Louis, Missouri: Elsevier Saunders.

PHOTO CREDITS

http://www.raymondhuber.co.nz/wp-content/uploads/2010/01/worker.jpg

http://static.vectorcharacters.net/uploads/2013/02/Young_Businesswoman_Vector_Character_Preview.jpg

http://ishmam.files.wordpress.com/2011/02/p540097-human_pancreas-spl.jpg

http://biology-forums.com/gallery/14755_14_10_12_6_35_06_93862089.jpeg

http://www.hivandhepatitis.com/0_images2009/cirrhosis2.jpg

http://upload.wikimedia.org/wikipedia/commons/thumb/9/98/Diagram_showing_fluid_(ascites)_being_drained_from_the_abdomen_CRUK_122.svg/2000px-Diagram_showing_fluid_(ascites)_being_drained_from_the_abdomen_CRUK_122.svg.png

https://www.itriagehealth.com/https_image_proxy?url=http%3A%2F%2Fs3.amazonaws.com%2Fitriage%2Fsourced%2Fsourced_images%2F288%2Foriginal.jpg%3F1370562799

http://4.bp.blogspot.com/-18UVLQKz7Rw/TtYRWNDf_tI/AAAAAAAAE50/kswgBB8SzUg/s320/2489.png

http://education-portal.com/cimages/multimages/16/esophageal_varices.jpg

http://www.ulcerativecolitis.net/wp-content/uploads/ulcerative-colitis.jpg

http://bionews-tx.com/wp-content/uploads/2013/10/crohns_disease.jpg

http://2.bp.blogspot.com/-UxLia61ukIo/T0MsQABskqI/AAAAAAAAAEA/bhLCDtpqSCE/s1600/main3.jpg

http://www.moondragon.org/health/graphics/appendicitis.jpg

http://www.physio-pedia.com/images/e/ed/Peptic-ulcers-lg-enlg.jpg

http://www.woyoso.org/images/hiatabeforeafter.jpg

http://2.bp.blogspot.com/-2_ZbhqWI6nQ/TrKy5YVZpPI/AAAAAAAADkY/tg-fCPGhQHo/s1600/toilet_cartoon_art_drawings_.jpg

http://pharmrx.yolasite.com/resources/ppn.jpg?timestamp=1278889989481

http://d26ua9paks4zq.cloudfront.net/78/a1/0651b2064703980466e4bb30eb93/BariumEnema_ORIGINAL_460x261.jpg

http://www.beverlyoakssurgery.com/wp-content/uploads/2012/04/endoscopy.jpg

http://www.hivandhepatitis.com/0_images_2008/liver_biopsy.gif

http://www.buildfire.com